RAPID ABG INTERPRETATION

BiPAP & Ventilator Handbook For MDs, RRTs, & RNs

Desmond Allen, PhD, RCP

Desmond Allen
Opelika, AL

© 2014 Create Space

ISBN-13: 978-1503304895

ISBN-10: 1503304892

PRINTED IN THE UNITED STATES OF AMERICA

Preface

I never cease to be amazed at the many clinicians confused by Arterial Blood Gas interpretation. In my experience, over the last couple decades this confusion has only grown worse, so that it is now endemic at all levels of healthcare professionals, from physicians to nurses and even some respiratory therapists.

I have determined the problem is not so much the students but the method by which they have been instructed to interpret ABGs. Thus, the objective of this booklet is to offer a simple and rapid method for ABG interpretation.

That being said, this is written specifically for those who have at least a cursory knowledge of the biochemistry and testing processes that constitute Arterial Blood Gas results: the Henderson–Hasselbalch equation, the Van Slyke method, the oxyhemoglobin dissociation curve, etc. As such, this work will not unduly rehearse these fundamental issues; at the same time, neither will it employ them to achieve our goal of rapid ABG interpretations. However, if the reader lacks knowledge of such fundamentals, certain terms and concepts might have little meaning.

Following rapid ABG interpretation our attention then turns to the treatment of various ventilatory and oxygenation abnormalities by the initiation and management of non-invasive pressure ventilation (generally referred to as Bilevel Positive Airway Pressure, or BiPAP) and to the more critical and invasive procedure of mechanical ventilation.

Table of Contents

CHAPTER THREE
CONCERNING OXYGENATION

SECTION TWO MECHANICAL INTERVENTION

CHAPTER FOUR
BIPAP SETTINGS AND MAINTENANCE

CHAPTER FIVE
BASIC VENTILATOR MANAGEMENT

CHAPTER SEVEN
ARDS/ALI VENTILATOR MANAGEMENT

CHAPTER EIGHT
VENTILATOR WEANING

Introduction

The rapid interpretation of ABGs need not be the ominous task that it is for so many. Herein, clinicians will learn to interpret ABGs rapidly by answering three simple questions.

- ✓ Is the pH normal, acidotic or alkalotic?

- ✓ Is the pH correctly predicted by the $PaCO_2$?

- ✓ If the pH is abnormal, is the abnormality caused, compensated or exacerbated by the $PaCO_2$?

By answering these simple questions we have all the information we need for an accurate interpretation—whether the ABG is normal, respiratory or metabolic acidosis, alkalosis, or both, acute, compensated or partially compensated.

Section One
Rapid ABG
Interpretation

Chapter One
ABG Interpretation Simplified

Arterial Blood Gases measure three values: ph, $PaCO_2$ and PaO_2; all other reported values are calculated from these three measurements. Thus, it is from these three basic values that we learn two sets of data: oxygenation and acid/base balance. If the ABG machine has a co-oximeter the oxygen saturation is measured, otherwise it too is merely calculated. Some ABG machines measure the electrolytes, but these values are technically not part of the ABG measurement; nor (as important as they may be to identifying certain conditions) are they involved in the rapid interpretation of ABG results.

The Acid/Base Confusion

The interpretation of oxygenation is relatively simple and will be discussed later; the confusion however, arises concerning interpretation of the acid/base balance aspects of ABGs. Here, I believe, the problem is not so much the student but the methods generally employed to instruct these students. Through the years several techniques have been imagined to help students interpret ABGs: arrows pointing up and down for various values, the likening of these values to family feuds, kissing cousins, black sheep, etc. However, the necessary employment of all such rote memory techniques suggests a failure to fully understand the fundamentals of acid/base balance, and thus continued confusion. Understanding the fundamentals of any subject is always better than rote memory. Understanding the fundamentals is a foundation upon which to build; mere rote memory allows for and enables confusion.

Perhaps the most confusing method, and one which seems to have gained popularity in recent decades, is the unwarranted attention given to the academic calculation of the bicarbonate (HCO_3-), and then using this calculated value as the primary factor to interpret ABGs. Although an interesting academic exercise, unfortunately this method merely confuses the matter of rapid ABG interpretation. Firstly, because most clinical practitioners (be they physicians, nurses or respiratory therapists) never fully master the biochemical processes nor the mathematical formulas concerning HCO_3-. Secondly, because HCO_3- is a calculated value (derived from the relationship between pH and $PaCO_2$) used primarily to arrive at yet another calculated value, the anion gap, which ironically, is a reported laboratory value aside from the ABG. Thirdly, because the anion gap is used to distinguish between various causes of metabolic adidosis, it is largely academic, in that the clinician likely already knows what is causing the acidosis. And finally, because this complicated method of highlighting a calculated value as the primary value by which to begin the interpretation process is completely unnecessary.

Rapid Acid/Base Balance Interpretation

Here, we shall see that everything we need to interpret the acid/base aspects of ABGs (so that immediate life support measures might be provided) is understood by the pH and $PaCO_2$. Anion gap issues, though potentially important, are a different concern than that of rapid ABG interpretation.

The objective of rapid ABG interpretation is to quickly and accurately differentiate between various clinical conditions so that rapid intervention, if necessary, can be employed. As such, we seek to determine such conditions as normal, acute respiratory and/or metabolic acidosis or alkalosis, compensated (chronic) or partially compensated respiratory or metabolic acidosis or alkalosis. All of these we will determine from two values, the pH and the $PaCO_2$.

Acid/Base Simplified

For the rapid interpretation of ABGs, we ask three simple questions and apply three simple rules. The answers to these questions and the application of these rules provide the interpretation.

Question #1
Is the pH normal, acidotic or alkalotic?

Question #2

Is the pH correctly predicted by the $PaCO_2$?

Question #3 - (ask only if answer to question #2 is No)

Is the abnormal pH caused, compensated or exacerbated by the $PaCO_2$?[1]

Rule #1

A change in $PaCO_2$ predicts a corresponding change in pH.

Rule #2

Any deviation from the predicted pH necessitates metabolic processes.[2]

Rule #3

The extent of metabolic involvement is determined by the degree to which the $PaCO_2$ fails to predict the pH.

	Normal	Normal Range
pH	= 7.40	(+/- 0.5) = 7.35 to 7.45

$PaCO_2$ = 40 mm Hg (+/- 0.5) = 35 to 45 mm Hg

---

[1] It should be noted complete compensation generally does not occur.

[2] Any metabolic involvement that is causing, exacerbating or compensating the abnormality is reflected in the calculated values of the HCO_3- and BE.

Chapter Two
Predicted Parameters

Rule #1 predicts a change in pH that corresponds directly to a change in $PaCO_2$. As such, increased $PaCO_2$ (which translates into increased acid) predicts a decreased or acidic pH. Conversely, decreased $PaCO_2$ (which translates into decreased acid) predicts an elevated or alkalotic pH. The predicted pH change is proportional to the actual change in $PaCO_2$. This predicted ratio is precise.

$$\Delta PaCO_2 \ 1 \text{ mm Hg} = \Delta \text{ pH } 0.00833$$

This a 12 to 0.1 ratio, thus:

$$\Delta 12 \ PaCO_2 \text{ mm Hg} = \Delta \text{ pH } 0.1$$

For example, a $PaCO_2$ of 40 mm Hg predicts a pH of 7.40. A $PaCO_2$ of 52 mm Hg (12 mm Hg higher than the normal 40 mm Hg) predicts a pH of 7.30, a corresponding acidic change in pH of 0.1 from the normal 7.40. Conversely, a $PaCO_2$ of 28 mm Hg (12 mm Hg below the normal 40 mm Hg) predicts a pH of 7.50, a corresponding alkalotic change of 0.1 from the normal 7.40.

The following table demonstrates this concept. However, this table need not be memorized; for once the 12 to 0.1 ratio (or 1 to 0.083) is understood predictions are easily calculated.

Actual PaCO$_2$	Δ	Predicted[3] pH
40	**0**	**7.40**
41	1	7.392
42	2	7.383
43	3	7.375
44	4	7.367
45	5	7.358
46	6	7.350
47	7	7.342
48	8	7.333
49	9	7.325
50	10	7.317
51	11	7.308
52	**12**	**7.30**
53	13	7.292
54	14	7.283
56	16	7.267
58	18	7.25
60	20	7.233
62	22	7.217
64	**24**	**7.2**
70	30	7.15
76	**36**	**7.1**

---

[3] 3rd decimal place given to clarify the math of 1 to 0.00833

Actual PaCO$_2$	Δ	Predicted pH
40	**0**	**7.40**
39	1	7.408
38	2	7.417
39	3	7.425
36	4	7.433
37	5	7.442
34	6	7.45
35	7	7.458
32	8	7.467
33	9	7.475
30	10	7.483
29	11	7.492
28	**12**	**7.50**
26	14	7.517
24	16	7.533
22	18	7.550
20	20	7.567
18	22	7.583
16	**24**	**7.60**
10	26	7.617
4	30	7.633

Application

Armed with these three questions and three rules, let's apply them to several examples and determine whether the ABG is normal, acute respiratory acidosis, acute respiratory alkalosis,

21

respiratory and metabolic acidosis or alkalosis, compensated (chronic) or partially compensated respiratory or metabolic acidosis or alkalosis.

Example #1:   Ph 7.40   PaCO₂ 40 mm Hg

Question #1
Is the pH normal, acidotic or alkalotic?

Answer: Normal.

Interpretation: Normal.

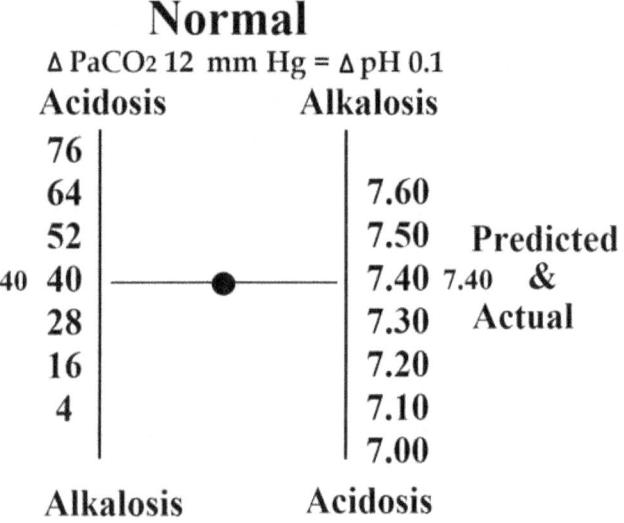

Normal

Δ PaCO$_2$ 12 mm Hg = Δ pH 0.1

Acidosis	Alkalosis
76	
64	7.60
52	7.50 Predicted
40 40	7.40 7.40 &
28	7.30 Actual
16	7.20
4	7.10
	7.00
Alkalosis	**Acidosis**

Example #2:   Ph 7.30   PaCO₂ 52 mm Hg

Question #1
Is the pH normal, acidotic or alkalotic?

Answer: Acidotic

Question #2
Is the pH correctly predicted by the $PaCO_2$?

Answer: Yes, the $PaCO_2$ 52 mm Hg predicts acidotic pH 7.30

Interpretation: Acute Respiratory Acidosis. The abnormal pH is completely accounted for by the abnormal $PaCO_2$; thus the acidosis is purely respiratory in origin.

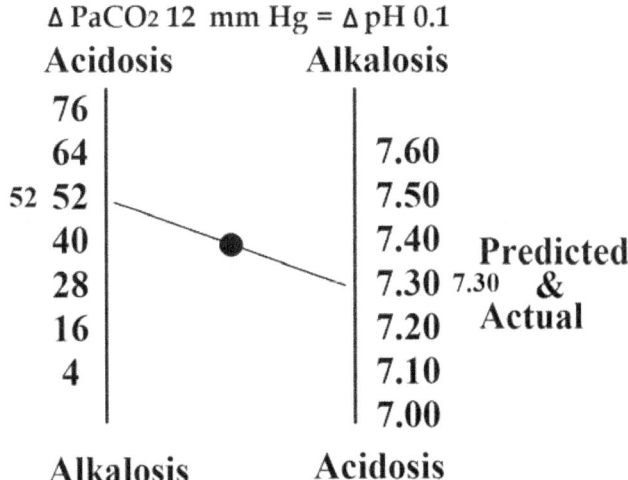

Acute Resp Acidosis
Δ PaCO₂ 12 mm Hg = Δ pH 0.1
Acidosis   Alkalosis

76
64   7.60
52 52   7.50
40   7.40   **Predicted**
28   7.30 7.30 **&**
16   7.20   **Actual**
4   7.10
              7.00
Alkalosis   Acidosis

Example #4:   Ph 7.25   PaCO$_2$ 58 mm Hg

Question #1
Is the pH normal, acidotic or alkalotic?

Answer: Acidotic.

Question #2
Is the pH correctly predicted by the PaCO$_2$?

Answer: Yes, PaCO$_2$ 58 mm Hg predicts acidosis pH 7.25.

Interpretation: Acute Respiratory Acidosis. The abnormal pH is completely accounted for by the abnormal PaCO$_2$; thus the acidosis is purely respiratory in origin.

Acute Resp Acidosis

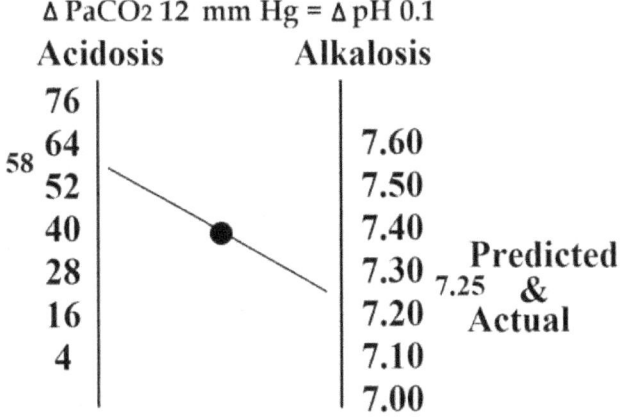

Δ PaCO2 12 mm Hg = Δ pH 0.1

Example #4:   Ph 7.30   PaCO$_2$ 40 mm Hg

Question #1
Is the pH normal, acidotic or alkalotic?

Answer: Acidotic.

Question #2
Is the pH correctly predicted by the PaCO$_2$?

Answer: No, PaCO$_2$ 40 mm Hg predicts a normal pH 7.40.

Question #3
Is the abnormal pH caused, compensated or exacerbated by the PaCO$_2$?

Answer: No, therefore it is completely metabolic.

25

Interpretation: Acute Metabolic Acidosis. There is no causative, compensating or exacerbating respiratory component involved.

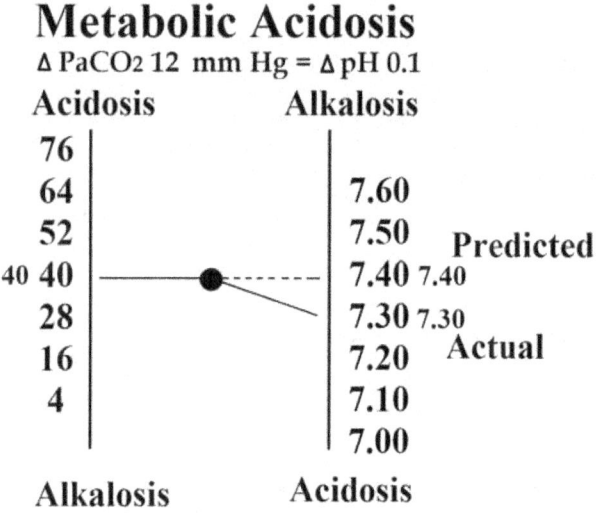

Metabolic Acidosis

$\Delta PaCO_2$ 12 mm Hg = ΔpH 0.1

Acidosis	Alkalosis
76	
64	7.60
52	7.50 Predicted
40 40	7.40 7.40
28	7.30 7.30
16	7.20 Actual
4	7.10
	7.00
Alkalosis	**Acidosis**

Example #5:   Ph 7.10   PaCO₂ 34 mm Hg

Question #1
Is the pH normal, acidotic or alkalotic?

Answer: Acidotic.

Question #2
Is the pH correctly predicted by the $PaCO_2$?

Answer: No, $PaCO_2$ 40 mm Hg predicts a normal pH 7.40.

Question #3
Is the abnormal pH caused, compensated or exacerbated by the $PaCO_2$?

Answer: No, therefore it is completely metabolic.

Interpretation: Metabolic Acidosis. There is no causative or exacerbating respiratory component involved; however the $PaCO_2$ 34 mm Hg shows that respiratory compensation is making an effort.

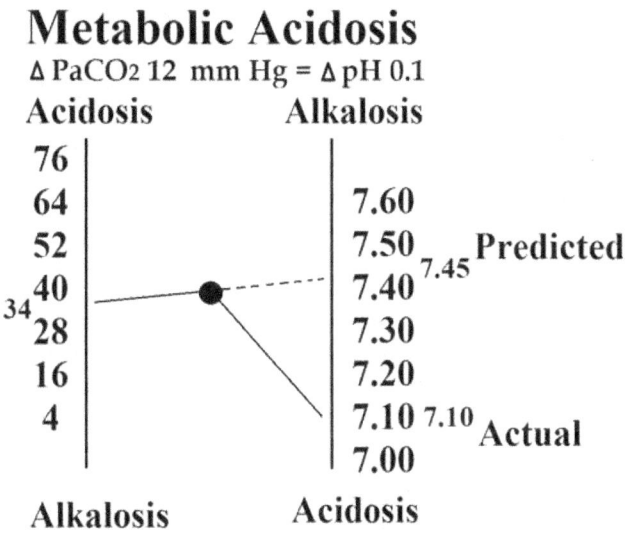

Metabolic Acidosis
Δ $PaCO_2$ 12 mm Hg = Δ pH 0.1

Example #6: Ph 7.35 $PaCO_2$ 64 mm Hg

Question #1

Is the pH normal, acidotic or alkalotic?

Answer: Acidotic.

Question #2

Is the pH correctly predicted by the $PaCO_2$?

Answer: No, $PaCO_2$ 64 mm Hg predicts an acidotic pH 7.20.

Question #3

Is the abnormal pH caused, compensated or exacerbated by the $PaCO_2$?

Answer: Yes, $PaCO_2$ 64 mm Hg predicts an acidotic pH 7.20, therefore pH 7.35 is being compensated by metabolic processes.

Interpretation: Compensated Respiratory Acidosis.

Compensated Resp Acidosis

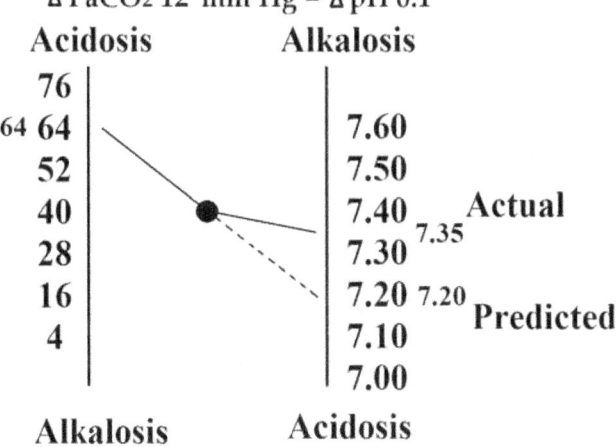

Δ PaCO₂ 12 mm Hg = Δ pH 0.1

Example #7: Ph 7.30 PaCO₂ 64 mm Hg

Question #1
Is the pH normal, acidotic or alkalotic?

Answer: Acidotic.

Question #2
Is the pH correctly predicted by the PaCO₂?

Answer: No, PaCO₂ 64 mm Hg predicts an acidotic pH 7.20.

Question #3
Is the abnormal pH caused, compensated or exacerbated by the PaCO₂?

Answer: Yes, $PaCO_2$ 64 mm Hg predicts an acidotic pH 7.20; therefore pH 7.30 is a partial compensation by metabolic processes.

Interpretation: Partially Compensated Respiratory Acidosis.

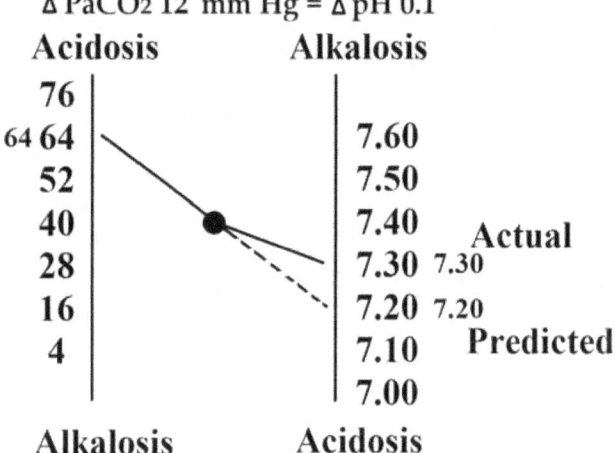

Part Comp Resp Acidosis
Δ $PaCO_2$ 12 mm Hg = Δ pH 0.1

Example #8: Ph 7.35 $PaCO_2$ 28 mm Hg

Question #1
Is the pH normal, acidotic or alkalotic?

Answer: Acidotic.

Question #2
Is the pH correctly predicted by the $PaCO_2$?

Answer: No, PaCO₂ 28 mm Hg predicts an alkalotic pH 7.50

Question #3
Is the abnormal pH caused, compensated or exacerbated by the PaCO₂?

Answer: An alkalotic PaCO₂ 28 mm Hg cannot cause of exacerbate an acidosis, therefore the acidotic pH 7.35 is metabolic and the alkalotic PaCO₂ 28 mm Hg is compensating for the metabolic acidosis.

Interpretation: Compensated Metabolic Acidosis.

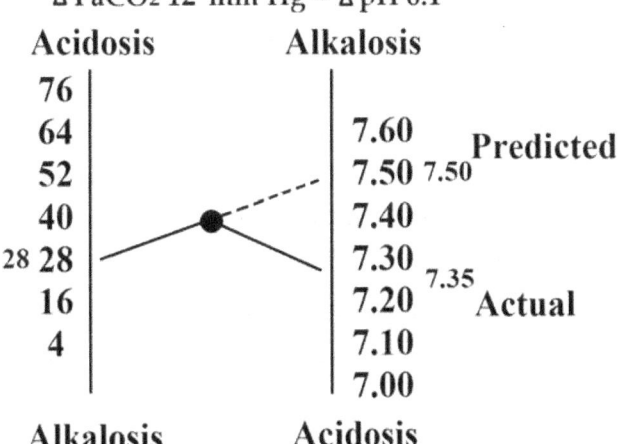

Comp Metabolic Acidosis
Δ PaCO2 12 mm Hg = Δ pH 0.1

Example #9: Ph 7.20   PaCO$_2$ 52 mm Hg

Question #1
Is the pH normal, acidotic or alkalotic?

Answer: Acidotic.

Question #2
Is the pH correctly predicted by the PaCO$_2$?

Answer: No, PaCO$_2$ 52 mm Hg predicts pH 7.30.

Question #3
Is the abnormal pH caused, compensated or exacerbated by the PaCO$_2$?

Answer: Yes, PaCO$_2$ 52 mm Hg predicts pH 7.30 thereby accounting for half of the acidosis; metabolic processes must account for the other half of the acidosis to achieve pH 7.20.

Interpretation: Respiratory and Metabolic Acidosis.

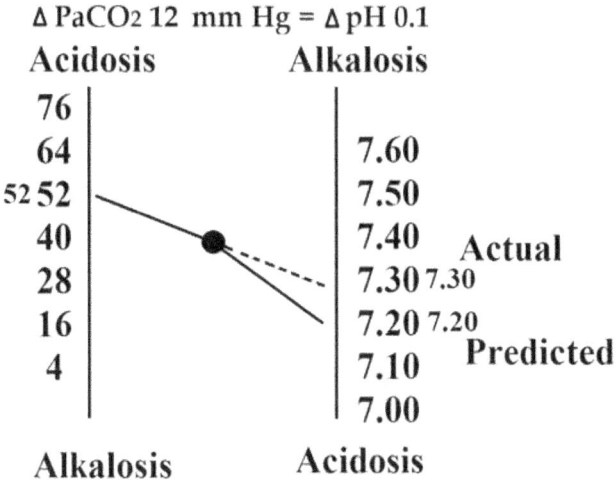

Resp & Met Acidosis

Δ PaCO2 12 mm Hg = Δ pH 0.1

Acidosis   **Alkalosis**

76	
64	7.60
52 52	7.50
40	7.40 **Actual**
28	7.30 7.30
16	7.20 7.20
4	7.10 **Predicted**
	7.00

Alkalosis   **Acidosis**

Example #10: Ph 7.50 PaCO$_2$ 28 mm Hg

Question #1
Is the pH normal, acidotic or alkalotic?

Answer: Alkalotic.

Question #2
Is the pH correctly predicted by the PaCO$_2$?

Answer: Yes, PaCO$_2$ 28 mm Hg predicts pH 7.50.

Interpretation: Acute Respiratory Alkalosis.

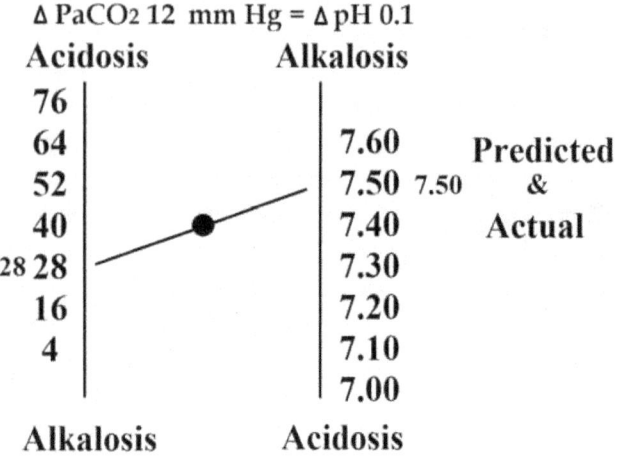

Acute Resp Alkalosis

Δ PaCO2 12 mm Hg = Δ pH 0.1

Example #11: Ph 7.52   PaCO$_2$ 46 mm Hg

Question #1
Is the pH normal, acidotic or alkalotic?

Answer: Alkalotic.

Question #2
Is the pH correctly predicted by the PaCO$_2$?

Answer: No, PaCO$_2$ 46 mm Hg predicts normal pH 7.35.

Question #3
Is the abnormal pH caused, compensated or exacerbated by the PaCO$_2$?

Answer: No, $PaCO_2$ 46 mm Hg predicts normal pH 7.35, therefore there is no respiratory involvement in the alkalosis; rather, $PaCO_2$ 46 mm Hg is beginning seeking to compensate for the metabolic Alkalosis.

Interpretation: Metabolic Alkalosis.

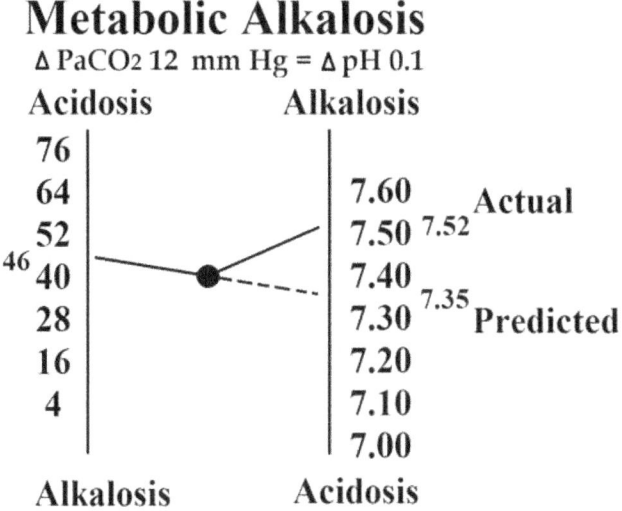

Metabolic Alkalosis
$\Delta\, PaCO_2$ 12 mm Hg = $\Delta\, pH$ 0.1

Example #12: Ph 7.48 $PaCO_2$ 22 mm Hg

Question #1
Is the pH normal, acidotic or alkalotic?

Answer: Alkalotic.

Question #2

35

Is the pH correctly predicted by the $PaCO_2$?

Answer: No, $PaCO_2$ 22 mm Hg predicts an alkalotic pH 7.55.

Question #3
Is the abnormal pH caused, compensated or exacerbated by the $PaCO_2$?

Answer: Yes, the $PaCO_2$ 22 mm Hg is the cause of the alkalotic pH 7.48. Because $PaCO_2$ 22 mm Hg predicts pH 7.55, the pH 7.48 is the result of partial compensation by metabolic processes.

Interpretation: Partially Compensated Respiratory Alkalosis.

Part Comp Resp Alkalosis

Δ $PaCO_2$ 12 mm Hg = Δ pH 0.1

Acidosis	Alkalosis

76	
64	7.60 Predicted
52	7.50 7.55
40	7.40 7.48
22 28	7.40 Actual
16	7.30
4	7.20
	7.10
	7.00

Alkalosis	Acidosis

Example #13:   Ph 7.45 $PaCO_2$ 52

Question #1
Is the pH normal, acidotic or alkalotic?

Answer: Alkalotic.

Question #2
Is the pH correctly predicted by the $PaCO_2$?
Answer: No, $PaCO_2$ 52 mm Hg predicts pH 7.30.

Question #3
Is the abnormal pH caused, compensated or exacerbated by the $PaCO_2$?

Answer: Yes, because $PaCO_2$ 52 mm Hg predicts an acidotic pH 7.30, the alkalotic pH 7.45 is due to metabolic processes; therefore $PaCO_2$ 52 mm Hg is compensating.

Interpretation: Compensated Metabolic Alkalosis.

Comp Met Alkalosis

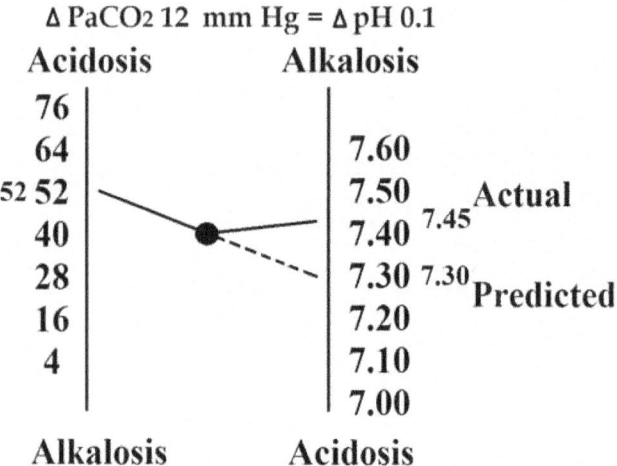

Δ PaCO2 12 mm Hg = Δ pH 0.1

Example #14: Ph 7.60   PaCO$_2$ 28 mm Hg

Question #1
Is the pH normal, acidotic or alkalotic?

Answer: Alkalotic.

Question #2
Is the pH correctly predicted by the PaCO$_2$?

Answer: No, PaCO$_2$ 28 mm Hg predicts pH 7.50.

Question #3

Is the abnormal pH caused, compensated or exacerbated by the $PaCO_2$?

Answer: Yes, because $PaCO_2$ 28 mm Hg predicts pH 7.50, it exacerbates the alkalosis but it does not account for the entirety of the alkalosis; therefore metabolic processes are also involved.

Interpretation: Respiratory and Metabolic Alkalosis.

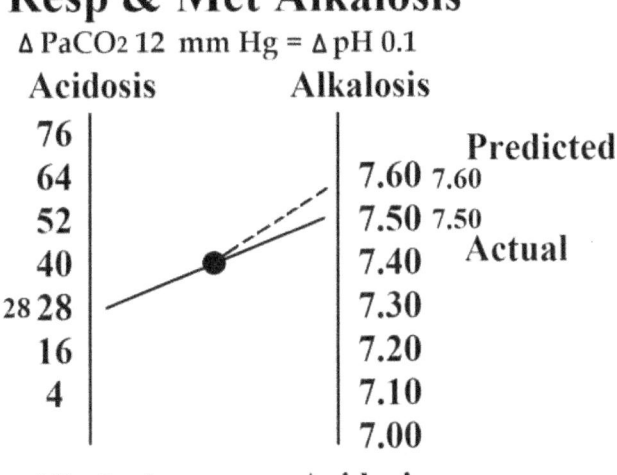

Resp & Met Alkalosis
$\Delta PaCO_2$ 12 mm Hg = Δ pH 0.1

Further Considerations

Similar to the proportional and predicted change in pH to changes in $PaCO_2$ (i.e. $PaCO_2$ 12 mm Hg predicts Δ pH 0.1), a corresponding and proportion change in the HCO_3- and BE occurs any time the pH fails to correspond to the $PaCO_2$ prediction.

This change reflects the degree of metabolic involvement.[4] So that, that portion of an abnormal pH for which the $PaCO_2$ fails to give account will be reflected by a corresponding change in HCO_3- and BE; each of which will vary slightly, depending on the acute versus chronic condition.

Because calculating the HCO_3- is far more involved than is the simple calculation of the BE, for rapid interpretation we shall simply consider the BE. Each change in pH of 0.1 (which is unaccounted for or unpredicted by the $PaCO_2$) will be reflected by a change in BE of roughly 6 mEq/L. Again, this is a rough estimate in that the BE and

---

[4] HCO_3- and BE are calculated values derived from the relationship between pH and $PaCO_2$; so that, while they are not necessary to ABG interpretation, neither are they without value. The HCO_3- is used to calculate the anion gap, which (by knowing if it is high, normal, or low) may help to narrow down the origin of a particular metabolic acidosis. Yet, on the other hand, even this is largely academic data; for the clinician will likely know what is causing the acidosis based upon the patient's condition — for example, DKA vs hemorrhage. Furthermore, the anion gap is reported by laboratory values so that this calculation is no longer necessary; which calculation by the way requires the serum concentration values for chloride, sodium and potassium. Clearly this is not the objective in rapid ABG interpretation within the average clinical setting. Nevertheless, the normal values for HCO_3- and BE are:

	Normal	Normal Range
HCO_3-	= 24 mEq/L	(+/- 2) = 22 to 26 mEq/L
BE	= 0 mEq/L	(+/- 2) = +2 to -2 mEq/L

HCO_3- can vary slightly, due to the acute versus chronic state. The change is less pronounced in acute conditions. Thus, the table of change is as such:

$$\Delta\, PaCO_2\ 12\ mm\ Hg = \Delta\, pH\ 0.1 = \Delta\, BE\ 6\ mEq/L$$

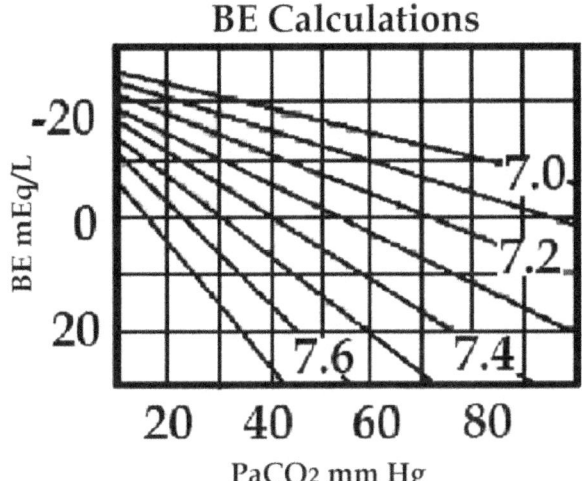

BE Calculations

$$\Delta\, PaCO_2\ 12\ mm\ Hg = \Delta\, pH\ 0.1 = \Delta\, BE\ 6\ mEq/L$$

Applying this detail we have examples such as the following. Keep in mind that BE values can very +/- 2 mEq/L depending upon the acute/chronic condition.

pH	PaCO$_2$	BE	Interpretation
7.40	40	0	Normal
7.30	52	0	Acute Respiratory Acidosis
7.30	42	-6	Acute Metabolic Acidosis
7.35	52	3	Compensated Resp Acidosis

7.35	34	-3	Comp Metabolic Acidosis
7.20	52	-6	Resp and Metabolic Acidosis
7.50	28	0	Acute Respiratory Alkalosis
7.50	40	6	Acute Metabolic Alkalosis
7.45	28	-3	Comp Respiratory Alkalosis
7.45	46	3	Comp Metabolic Alkalosis
7.60	28	6	Resp and Metabolic Alkalosis

The following graphs are replicas of those we looked at earlier; however, these include the calculated Base Excess.

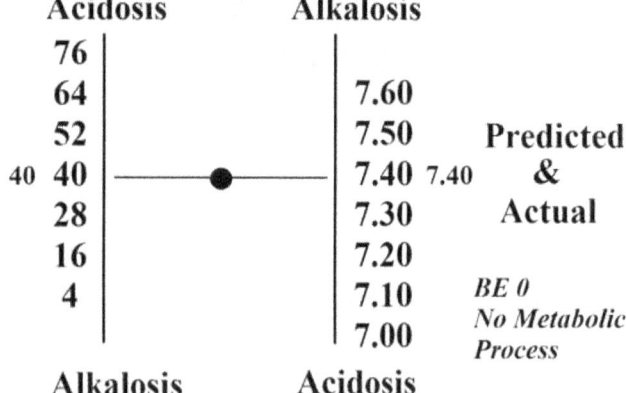

Normal

Δ PaCO2 12 mm Hg = Δ pH 0.1 = Δ BE 6 mEq/L

Acute Resp Acidosis

Δ PaCO₂ 12 mm Hg = Δ pH 0.1 = Δ BE 6 mEq/L

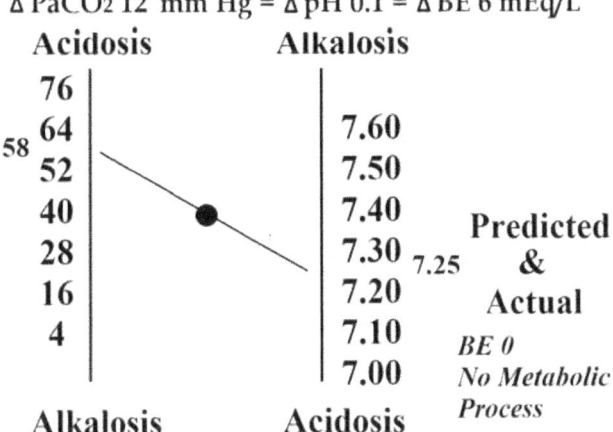

Compensated Resp Acidosis

Δ PaCO₂ 12 mm Hg = Δ pH 0.1 = Δ BE 6 mEq/L

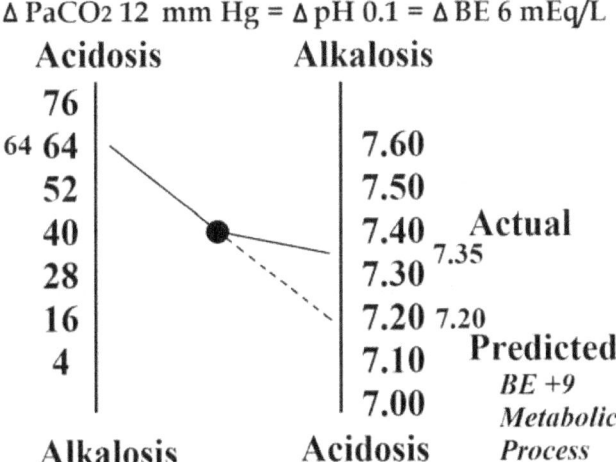

Comp Metabolic Acidosis

Δ PaCO2 12 mm Hg = Δ pH 0.1 = Δ BE 6 mEq/L

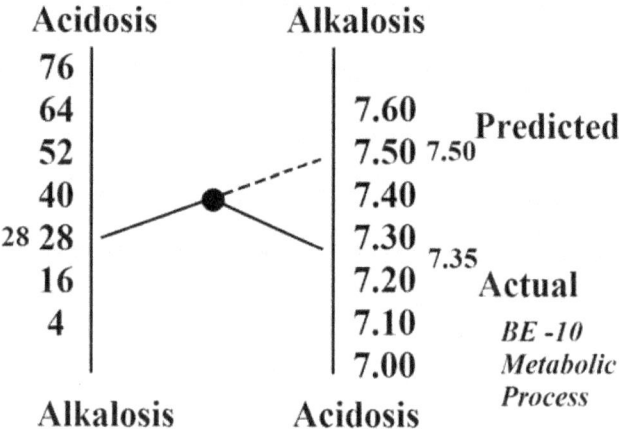

Chapter Three
Concerning Oxygenation

Understanding the concept of oxygenation, as reflected in the ABG, is seldom an issue; it is rather straight forward. However, accurately treating various hypoxemic conditions can be more of a challenge. Normal PaO_2 is 80 to 100 mg Hg. A PaO_2 below 80 mm Hg is considered hypoxemia. A normal SaO_2 is considered to 90% to 100%. But there are a few caveats:

- Saturation values as low as 88% are generally considered acceptable in severe COPD patients.

- A primary hemoglobin deficiency, such as anemia, is typically not considered a cause of hypoxemia.

- CO poisoning will mask an abnormal SaO_2.

- Hypoxemia of PaO_2 60 mm Hg or lower with FiO_2 60% or greater is considered refractory hypoxemia and (barring anemia or CO poisoning) is generally due to ventilation/perfusion imbalances. For this, intervention beyond mere supplemental oxygen (such as diuretic, dialysis, BiPAP and or intubation and mechanical ventilation) is generally required.

Various Causes of Hypoxemia

■ Low inspired partial pressure of oxygen (PIO_2). *Due to anesthesia, or low barometric pressure such as in high altitude.*

■ Alveolar hypoventilation. *Due to airway obstruction, CNS depression, or muscular weakness.*

■ Impaired diffusion across capillary/blood-gas membrane. *Such as alveolar fibrosis (rare).*

■ Increased systemic oxygen consumption. *Due to fever, exertion, acidosis, etc*

■ Ventilation/Perfusion imbalances. *Account for 95% of abnormal gas exchange. Cardiogenic shunts cannot be corrected with 100% FiO_2; some pulmonary shunts can be.*

■ Hypoxemia: PaO_2 < 60 mmHg. *Typically responds well to supplemental oxygen adjusted to maintain a SpO_2 of 90% or greater. Exceptions are low hemoglobin or CO poisoning.*

Oxyhemoglobin Dissociation Curve

Having a basic understanding of the oxyhemoglobin dissociation curve is necessary to adequately assess and thus properly maintain appropriate FiO_2 and SaO_2. Although, as stated earlier, it is not the objective of this work to explain fundamentals, let's rehearse a few of the basics. The ODC is an XY graphic portrayal of PaO_2 and SaO_2 in relation to pH; wherein it expresses the hemoglobin's affinity for oxygen molecules—how readily hemoglobin receives or binds with oxygen and conversely releases oxygen to peripheral tissues. This affinity is affected by pH, carbon dioxide content $P(CO_2)$ and temperature.

As its partial pressure increases, oxygen molecules readily bind to the hemoglobin, as indicated by the initial steep portion of the ODC. As maximum saturation is approached (especially at pressures above 60 mm Hg) binding grows proportionally less in respect increased $FiO2$ concentrations, as indicated by the flatter portion of the curve. The p50 (at which point the hemoglobin is 50% saturated) generally marks the divide between the primarily upwardly steep and more flattening portions of the ODC and is used to indicate a right or left shift, which (if present) occurs due to changes in $P(CO_2)$, temperature or pH.

A decreased $P(CO_2)$ or temperature, or an increased pH is reflected by a left shift of the curve and results in the hemoglobin's enhanced affinity for oxygen molecules. As such, it more easily accepts oxygen but then does not release it to the tissue with similar ease. Conversely, an increased $P(CO_2)$ or temperature, or a decrease pH is reflected by a right shift in the curve and results in the hemoglobin's decreased affinity for oxygen molecules. As such, it less easily accepts oxygen but then also releases the oxygen to the tissue with greater ease.

In simple terms, the more alkalotic the pH, or the lower the temperature, the greater the hemoglobin binds to oxygen molecules, thus it easily accepts the oxygen but then does not release it to the tissue with similar ease. The more acidotic the pH, or the higher the temperature, the more the opposite affect occurs—the hemoglobin binds less easily with the oxygen but then also releases it to the tissue more easily.

With this understanding we know that an ODC shift to the right requires a greater PaO_2 in order to achieve the same SaO_2 that would be achieved with a normal pH and thus a normal curve; therefore, an increased FiO_2 or PEEP is often required.

Oxygen Dissociation Curve

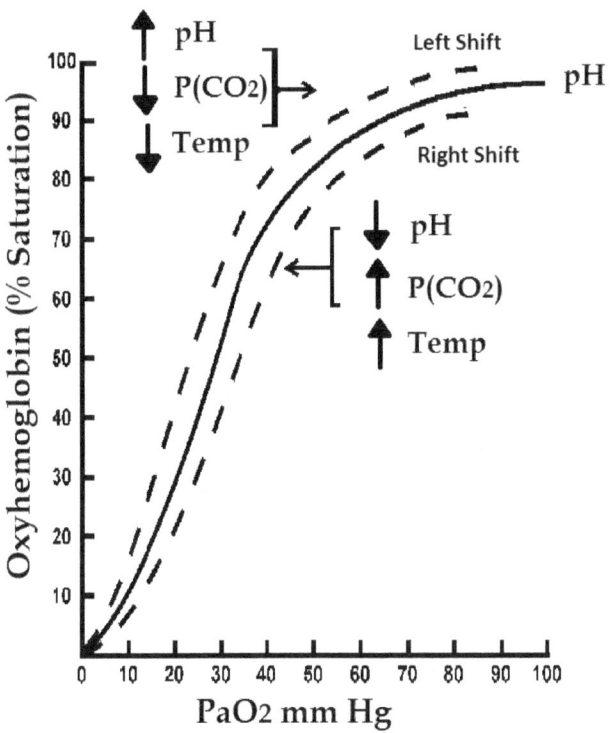

Quick SaO$_2$ & PaO$_2$ Assessment

Based upon the oxyhemoglobin dissociation curve, and without actually obtaining an ABG, there is a helpful rule of thumb used to estimate PaO$_2$ from the known SaO$_2$. This is especially useful once the patient's baseline PaCO$_2$/SaO$_2$ has been established with an ABG. For patients on mechanical ventilation, monitored by SpO$_2$ and End-Tidal CO$_2$ (ETCO$_2$), which have also been correlated to a baseline ABG, this rule of thumb can help diminish the number of unnecessary ABGs.

4-5-6, 7-8-9 Rule of Thumb

PaO_2 **40**% = SaO_2 is **7**0%

PaO_2 **50**% = SaO_2 is **8**0%

PaO_2 **60**% = SaO_2 is **9**0%

Caveats

This assumes the patient is less than 60, is not a chronic CO_2 retainer, and that the pH is within normal limits. In which cases small adjustments must be made.

Section Two
Mechanical
Intervention

Chapter Four
BiPAP Settings and Maintenance

Because ventilatory changes are often necessary on a dynamic basis, for best results, it is suggested that the implementation of the following guidelines transcend the solely physician driven approach; thereby, to some degree, incorporating the entire critical care team: physicians, respiratory care practitioners, and registered nurses. It has been well established that using patient driven versus physician driven protocols reduces the time of mechanical ventilation, thereby having a positive affect on ventilator complications and ultimately reducing the length of stay.

The objective in this section is to facilitate the application, management, and timely discontinuation of BiPAP or CPAP therapies when used to treat respiratory failure or impending respiratory failure.

Definition of Terms

CPAP (Continuous Positive Airway Pressure) delivers a single, constant pressure during both inhalation and exhalation.

BiPAP (Bi-level Positive Airway Pressure) or *NPPV* (Noninvasive Positive Pressure Ventilation) delivers two pressures. The lesser pressure, referred to as ePAP (Expiratory Positive Airway Pressure), is delivered upon exhalation. The second and greater pressure, referred to as iPAP (Inspiratory Positive Airway Pressure), which is delivered during inhalation.

CPAP/ePAP & Acute Respiratory Failure

CPAP or ePAP is generally employed to achieve one of two objectives: (1) to splint the upper airway as a treatment for sleep apnea; or (2) to augment oxygenation in the presence of refractory hypoxemia (i.e. PaO2 < 60mm Hg, or SaO_2 < 90% with FiO_2 > 60%). Our concern in this work is with the second objective, the treatment of refractory hypoxemia. This form of respiratory failure is generally cased by a ventilation/perfusion mismatch; which is often observed in such conditions as CHF, atelectasis, pulmonary embolism and pneumonia.

CPAP or ePAP treats refractory hypoxemia by increasing and maintaining alveolar pressures, which in turn promotes alveolar recruitment and oxygen diffusion.

BiPAP & Acute Respiratory Failure

When respiratory failure or impending respiratory failure is solely a matter of refractory hypoxemia with no ventilatory compromise, and the patient is not yet to that critical point of intubation and volume ventilation, CPAP (or ePAP) and high FiO_2 concentrations are generally sufficient.

If ventilation is compromised, BiPAP could be the treatment of choice. Because iPAP augments ventilation, BiPAP can be an effective treatment for acute hypercapnia. COPD, multiple rib fractures with a flail segment or even extreme pain secondary to a post-operative incision are common causes of acute hypercapnia.

Because iPAP augments ventilation and ePAP augments oxygenation, BiPAP can be used to treat concurrent refractory hypoxemia and hypercapnia.

When treating acute hypercapnic respiratory failure, the distance between the iPAP and ePAP pressures is of primary importance with the ePAP often set at no more than 4 cm H_20. This is because ventilatory assistance increases as the distance between iPAP and ePAP widens. For example, an iPAP/ePAP of 16/4 provides greater ventilatory assistance than does 16/6.

When treating refractory hypoxemia it is the ePAP that is most crucial. Here, an iPAP/ePAP setting of 14/8 or even 12/8 would be more appropriate than the 16/4 used to initiate treatments for the hypercapnic patient.

If used to treat both refractory hypoxemia and hypercapnia simultaneously, we seek to achieve optimal ventilation via widening the iPAP and ePAP pressures, and optimal oxygenation via a higher ePAP pressure. Thus, something along the lines 16/8 or 18/8 would provide both ventiltory support and promote oxygenation. In either case, settings should be titrated for optimal affect and patient comfort.

Contraindications to CPAP/BiPAP Therapy

The following conditions are contraindicated for either CPAP or BiPAP therapy:

1. Patients with severe respiratory failure without a spontaneous respiratory drive.

2. Decreased level of consciousness that prevents the patient's ability to protect his/her own airway.

3. Inability to maintain a patent airway or adequately clear secretions.

4. Non-compliant patient.

In the following conditions, the risk versus benefit of ventilatory assistance should be carefully considered before employing CPAP/BiPAP therapy.

1. Risk for aspiration of gastric content. In such cases a NG tube can be helpful.

2. Bullous lung disease (emphysema).

3. Pre-existing pneumothroax or pneumomediastinum, which may be complicated due to increased pressure.

4. Hypotension.

5. Acute sinusitis or otitis media.

6. Epistaxis.

7. Recent facial, oral or skull surgery or trauma.

8. History of allergy or sensitivity to mask materials.

Potential Complications

1. Skin breakdown and discomfort from mask. While the initial skin integrity is an issue, breakdown is a virtually certainty for everyone after several days of continuous therapy.

2. Gastric distention.

3. Increased intracranial pressure.

4. Pulmonary barotraumas.

5. Cardiovascular compromise.

Selection of Therapy

To determine the therapeutic objective, consider the following questions. What is being treated: Acute hypercapnia? Refractory hypoxemia? Or both?

1. If refractory hypoxemia is the sole issue CPAP is the desired treatment. Here, ventilatory assistance is not an issue. As evidenced by ABGs, it is not uncommon for CHF patients suffering acute refractory hypoxemia to be hyperventilating. In such cases unnecessary ventilatory support will further decrease an already low $PaCO_2$.

2. If acute hypercapnia is the sole issue, BiPAP with a low ePAP setting is the desired

treatment; for here ventilation is the issue, while oxygenation augmentation is not.

3. If both refractory hypoxemia and acute hypercapnia are at issue, BiPAP with a higher ePAP pressure is the desired treatment; for here both ventilatory assistance and oxygenation augmentation are of concern.

BiPAP Settings

All settings are considered dynamic, in that they may need adjustment to meet patient demand as the condition changes. As such, the following suggested guidelines provide a standardized basis from which to initiate settings and make said changes.

CPAP/ePAP settings for Refractory Hypoxemia

1. FiO_2 100%.

2. CPAP/ePAP to 8 cm H_2O.

3. Increase/Decrease in increments of 2 cm H_2O, as tolerated, to maintain desired SaO_2 (e.g. > 90%).

4. If a CPAP/ePAP setting > 14 cm H_2O fails to maintain desired SaO_2, consider other options: additional pharmaceutical interventions, dialysis, increased pressure, or intubation and mechanical ventilation.

Management & Weaning from CPAP/ePAP

1. Decrease CPAP/ePAP in increments of 2 cm H_2O while maintaining desired SaO_2 as monitored by SpO_2.

2. Once desired SaO_2 is maintained at < 8 cm H_2O, periodically decrease FiO_2 by 10% increments while maintaining desired SaO_2.

3. Once FiO2 50% is achieved and desired SaO_2 is maintained, periodically decrease ePAP in increments of 2 cm H_2O as tolerated.

4. Once desired SaO_2 is maintained with FiO2 50% and CPAP/ePAP 4 cm H_2O, place patient on 50% venti-mask. If unable to maintain desired SaO_2, resume CPAP/ePAP at the lowest setting necessary to maintain SaO_2.

5. Attempt 50% venti-mask trials as tolerated.

BiPAP settings for Acute Hypercapnia

1. For acute hypercapnia, FiO_2 21% or > to maintain desired SaO_2 (e.g. ≥ 88% for known $PaCO_2$ retainers; 90% if refractory hypoxemia is also an issue; ≥ 92% for all others). If refractory hypoxemia is also an issue, use 100% as stated above under CPAP/ePAP settings for refractory hypoxemia.

2. Begin with ePAP 4 to 6 cm H20. If refractory hypoxemia is also an issue, begin at 8 cm H_20 as stated above under CPAP/ePAP settings for refractory hypoxemia.

3. Begin iPAP 6 to 12 cm H_2O above selected ePAP setting (e.g. 10/4, 14/6, 16/4, etc.). Ultimately, these setting might need titrating to achieve optimal ventilatory assistance, patient comfort and to address clinical factors: minute volume, respiratory rate, SaO_2, observed work of breathing, and ABGs if deemed necessary.

Management and Weaning from BiPAP

1. Incrementally increase/decrease iPAP by 2 cm H_2O while continuing to meet the patient's ventilatory needs as evidenced by patient comfort and clinical indications.

2. Incrementally increase/decrease FiO_2 to maintain desired SaO_2.

3. Once iPAP of $\leq$ 6 cm H_2O above ePAP is achieved with clinical signs remaining stable, attempt to remove BiPAP for short periods as tolerated. Place patient on an appropriate and adequate $Fi0_2$ source to maintain desire SaO_2 during these trials. Increase the duration and frequency of these trials as tolerated.

4. If refractory hypoxemia is also an issue, follow the ePAP weaning guidelines

described above before attempting BiPAP removal trials.

5. Immediately return patient to BiPAP upon any clinical signs of distress; such as failing to maintain SaO_2, markedly increased HR (> 20%), marked increased WOB, or patient-stated SOB/discomfort, etc.

Chapter Five
Basic Ventilator Management

The objective for the following guidelines is to provide a safe and efficient standardized approach to mechanical ventilation setup, management and weaning. The guidelines are based upon current technology, recent studies, and protocols as set forth by the American Association for Respiratory Care (AARC).

Even after initial settings have been selected, changes in the patient's condition or various problematic ventilatory issues (such as pressure limits, oxygenation, hemodynamic instability, patient discomfort, etc.,) might need immediate attention. Thus, the cookie cutter approach to ventilator settings is not acceptable; nor is it generally acceptable to have ventilator settings managed by a physician who is not at bedside. Therefore, it is best to have policies and procedure prepared that allow in-house physicians or respiratory therapists to manage the ventilator settings in real time. The following guidelines can provide much of the necessary data to construct such policies and procedures.

Definition of Modes

Mandatory Breath Modes

Volume Ventilation (VV): A preset volume is delivered in either the assist/control (AC) or command minute volume (CMV) mode, wherein every breath (whether by demand or patient generated) receives a set volume; or the Synchronized Intermittent Mandatory Ventilation (SIMV), wherein a set volume is delivered at a determined rate while any additional respirations are generated and regulated by the patient's own efforts, although pressure support can be added to augment the patient's ventilation.

Pressure Ventilation (PV) or pressure control ventilation (PCV): A preset pressure is delivered in either AC or SIMV.

Pressure Regulated Volume Control (PRVC): *[Note, this acronym and nomenclature may change from one ventilator manufacturer to another]*: A set pressure is automatically regulated throughout the inspiration to adjust for airway resistance as a determined volume is delivered. This mode is used in either AC, or SIMV.

Airway Pressure Release Ventilation (APRV): *[Note, this acronym and nomenclature may change from one ventilator manufacturer to another]*: A pressure ventilation in which inverse ratios are utilized via high pressure and low pressures.

Support Breath Modes

Pressure Support (PS): A patient-triggered, pressure targeted, flow-cycled mode. This can be a stand-alone breath in patients who have an intact respiratory drive, or used in combination with mandatory breath.

Volume Support (VS): A patient-triggered, pressure targeted, flow-cycled mode that guarantees a set volume. This can be a stand-alone breath in patients who have an intact respiratory drive, or used in combination with mandatory breath types.

Spontaneous Mode/CPAP: A solely patient driven rate, which allows for monitoring patient data, alarms, and baseline adjustment. PS and/or PEEP can be employed.

Mode Suggestions

As simplistic as it may sound, when choosing a mode of ventilation it is imperative to consider the specific reason for employing mechanical ventilation: CHF, COPD exacerbation, surgical recovery, hypoxemia due to pneumonia, etc., for these initial decisions often set the course for the next 24 or 48 hours. Beginning with the most appropriate mode and settings can lead to a more rapid and satisfactory weaning process. Or more accurately, beginning with an inappropriate mode can unduly delay the weaning process.

In the initial phase of acute respiratory failure, nearly total or even total ventilator support via a volume mode (AC or SIMV) is recommended. As the patient's condition improves other modes might be employed to allow varying degrees of spontaneous ventilatory activity to maintain diaphragm strength.

Things to Consider

For patient's moving a little or no minute volume, or conversely, those demanding excessive minute volumes, AC might be more appropriate. This will control the apneic or near apneic patient, and conversely, will ease the work of breathing (WOB) for the patient with a high minute volume demand, such as the septic patient.

For patients with an inadequate respiratory drive, in need of minimal or moderate support, SIMV volume ventilation might be more efficient. This assures an adequate minute volume while simultaneously allowing patient to control at least some portion of their tidal volumes.

Generally pressure support is employed to augment these spontaneous breaths or, at the very least, to overcome tube resistance so the patient does not feel as though he/she is breathing through a straw. About 5 cm H_2O will suffice to overcome tube resistance.

While this mode is generally used to decrease WOB, it can also be used to increase WOB. For example, if moving from AC (wherein WOB can be minimal) to SIMV (in which WOB requires more effort) we might purposely increase WOB to maintain diaphragmatic muscle tone.

Asthmatics are often more comfortable in pressure modes than volume modes, or in SIMV with PS and a low demand rate. Generally, other modes such as PRVC, APRV, PCV, PV, etc., might be employed to manage certain ventilation issues that might arise.

For example, other modes might be considered if peak pressures rise over 40 cm H_2O, or if plateau pressures (Pplateau) rise > 30 cm H_2O.

PS and PEEP in Spontaneous Ventilation mode can be effective in patients with a near adequate respiratory drive or who are weaning from tolerate ventilation support.

Ventilator Setup

To determine the initial tidal and minute volumes we must know or estimate the patient's ideal body weight, actual body surface area, consider the immediate clinical needs, and the patient's physical condition—for example is their only one lung.

Initial Tidle Volume

The initial V_T in any volume mode is based upon the patient's ideal body weight (IBW); thus, immediately, calculations are required. And, as mentioned earlier, a cookie cutter approach (such as men 700cc, women 600cc), which is all too often employed, is not sufficient.

Another common error is to calculate V_T based on the patient's actual weight. This often leads to unnecessarily large volumes, which is turn generates high airway pressures that can lead to barotrauma. Irregardless of one's actual weight, the lungs do not grow larger; thus V_T is calculated on IBW.

Target an initial V_T of 8 ml/kg IBW, while maintaining a Pplateau < 30 cm H_2O and delta P < 20 cm H2O. Based upon the patient's condition,

V_T adjustments may range from 4 to 12 ml/kg IBW to maintain the parameters of Pplateau < 30 cm H_2O and delta P < 20 cm H2O. Consult the pulmonologist if unable to maintain these parameters.

Calculating IBW

Males IBW (kg) = 50 + 2.3 kg for each inch over 60

Females IBW (kg) = 45.5 + 2.3 kg for each inch over 60

Initial Minute Volume

Minute volume, on the other hand, does increase as one's BSA increases, so that MV is based upon the patient's actual size; again, calculations are required. The targeted MV is achieved primarily by adjusting the respiratory rate once the V_T is determined, 8 to 26 breaths/minute are generally sufficient.

Then, if necessary small adjustments to V_T can be made as several factors permit: peak airway pressures (PIP), Pplateau < 30 cm H_2O, delta P < 20 cm H_2O, and maintaining an adequate I:E Ratio. Adjustments in respiratory rate and flow rate will determine the I:E Ratio, which should be set for optimum mean airway pressure, lung filling, exhalation (minimizing air-trapping/Auto-PEEP), and patient/ventilator synchrony.

Calculating BSA

BSA = [(Height{in} x Weight{lbs}) / (3131)] x 0.5

Males: BSA x 4.0 = V_E (L/min)

Female: BSA x 3.5 = V_E (L/min)

Reference Tables for V_T & MV

The following quick reference table for V_T is expressed in cc's and is calculated by 8 cm H_2O/kg of IBW.   Due to unknown variables that are particular to each patient, the quick reference table for targeted MV (expressed in liters) is based upon ideal BSA. However, an additional, modified MV, based upon 20% obesity, is also provided. Both V_T and MV for those patients lying outside of these tables (whether shorter, taller, or heavier) are easily extrapolated. Furthermore, these figures are merely projected starting points for which fine adjustments will likely be necessary once more data is acquired: ABGs, PIP, I:E Ratio, patient comfort, etc.

Males Actual Ht Inches	Target V_T	Target MV	20% Obese MV
61	418	4.48	5.38
62	437	4.76	5.71
63	455	5.04	6.05
64	474	5.32	6.39
65	492	5.62	6.74
66	510	5.92	7.10
67	538	6.22	7.47
68	547	6.54	7.84
69	566	6.86	8.23

70	584	7.18	8.62
72	621	7.85	9.42
73	639	8.20	9.84
74	658	8.55	10.26
75	676	8.91	10.69
76	694	9.27	11.12

Females Actual Ht Inches	Target V_T	Target MV	20% Obese MV
61	382	3.59	4.30
62	401	3.82	4.58
63	419	4.06	4.87
64	438	4.30	5.17
65	456	4.56	5.47
66	474	4.81	5.78
67	493	5.07	6.09
68	511	5.34	6.41
69	530	5.62	6.74
70	548	5.90	7.08
72	585	6.47	7.77
73	603	6.77	8.12
74	622	7.07	8.48
75	640	7.38	8.85
76	658	7.69	9.23

Oxygenation

The initial FiO_2 will vary widely depending upon the patient's condition and the reason for employing mechanical ventilation. Many post-op patients, or even patients suffering COPD exacerbation, may only need ventilation support and thus no more than a 25% or 30% FiO2, Many CHF patients, or others suffering refectory hypoxemia from a variety of medical conditions, will require no less than 100% FiO_2, and my need little to nor ventilation support. However, many patients will need both ventilation and oxygenation.

PEEP & PS

An initial PEEP is generally a minimum of 5 cm H_2O to emulate the anatomical PEEP provided by the epiglottis, which is now being bypassed by the entubation tube. Many clinicians will set 0 PEEP when the patient's blood pressure is dangerously low, so as not to further impede venous return. That being said, PEEP as high as 12 or even 20 cm H_2O may be required in ARDS or ALI. Other, less ominous conditions of ventilation/perfusion mismatch resulting in refectory hypoxemia might do very well at 8 cm H_2O PEEP. Beyond the emulation of anatomical PEEP, it is generally best to employ as little PEEP as necessary to accomplish the desired SaO_2.

Pressure Support (PS) is generally set from 5 to 20 cm H_2O. While 5 cm H_2O merely serves to overcome tube resistance so patient do not feel as though they are breathing through straws, larger pressures can significantly augment ventilation. However, when PS as high as 20 cm H_2O are required to meet patient demand, it might be best to consider increasing the frequency of volume ventilation.

Continued Ventilator Management

Once the mode of ventilation and settings are selected, subsequent and sometimes frequent adjustments are often required to achieve and maintain the desired parameters.

Initial ABG

Obtain an initial ABG about 30 to 60 minutes after mechanical ventilation begins and correlated both the SpO_2 and $ETCO_2$ with the SaO_2 and $PaCO_2$ values. Adjust the ventilator settings to achieve and maintain acceptable ABG results for the following patient categories.

Category	pH	$PaCO_2$	PaO_2	SpO_2
Normal	7.35-7.45	35 - 45	> 80	92-97%
CO_2 Retainer	7.30-7.45	45 - 55	55 - 75	> 89%
ALI/ARDS	7.25-7.45	Maintain pH	> 60	90-95%

Once the initial tidle volume and minute volume have been established via the previous mentioned guidelines, fine adjustments might be required. The SpO_2 and $ETCO_2$ can be used to predict and target the desired pH and PaO_2. As the pH or temperature changes, or the metabolic components normalize or are corrected medically the SpO_2/$ETCO_2$/ABG correlation may need to be reestablished.

Minute Volume Parameters

For pH < 7.30, incrementally adjust the rate (to a maximum of 26) over the first hour attempting to achieve a pH > 7.30. If further adjustment is needed, incrementally increase V_T until PIP = 40 cm H_2O or Pplateau = 30 cm H^2O. If these adjustments are unable to achieve and maintain a desired pH within said parameters, consult the pulmonologist and consider permissive hypercapnia.

In conditions of respiratory alkalosis (such as persistent hypoxemia with a resultant, which fails to respond to high PEEP and 100% FiO_2), adjust the rate (to a minimum of 8 breaths/minute) seeking to achieve a pH < 7.45. Again, a specific $ETCO_2$ can be targeted that will predict the desired pH. If further adjustments are required, reduce volume to a minimum of 4 ml/kg IBW.

Oxygenation Parameters

Consult the pulmonologist and consider following an ARDS/ALI protocol if the following limitations are crossed: PaO_2/FiO_2 ratio is ≤ 300, or FiO_2 50% and PEEP 12 cm H_2O are insufficient to maintain appropriate oxygenation.

Although the SpO_2 is being monitored to assure an adequate PaO_2 is achieved, hemoglobin should be checked to ensure the absence of anemia, and hemodynamic data monitored to ensure the potential for adequate perfusion. Consider inserting an A-Line if more than one ABG per day is required or anticipated.

Chapter Seven
ARDS/ALI Ventilator Management

Mechanical ventilation of patients with Acute Respiratory Distress Syndrome (ARDS) or Acute Lung Injury (ALI) centers on peak airway and plateau pressures. However, the following basic guidelines may not be appropriate for patients with conditions in which hypercapnia would not be tolerated (e.g. raised intracranial pressure, spinal cord injury, tricyclic antidepressant overdose, sickle cell disease). As always, if uncertainty exists, consult the pulmonologist.

ARDS/ALI Inclusion Criteria

The following ARDS/ALI basic guidelines are recommended in the presence of the following criteria.

- PaO_2/FiO_2 ratio is ≤ 300, or setting of FiO_2 50% and PEEP 12 cm H_2O are insufficient to maintain appropriate oxygenation.

- Radiographic images of bilateral (patchy, diffuse, or homogeneous) infiltrates consistent with pulmonary edema.

- No clinical evidence of left atrial hypertension.

Tidal Volume

For ventilator management in ARDS/ALI it is deemed critical to maintain low peak airway pressures; thus, if in a volume ventilation mode, low tidal volumes are employed. So that (unless the current V_T is lower than 8 ml/kg IBW), begin with V_T of 8 ml/kg IBW.

- Reduce V_T by 1 ml/kg at intervals $\leq$ 2 hours until V_T = 6ml/kg IBW.

- If necessary, repeat this process to a minimal V_T of 4 ml/kg IBW.

- If a V_T of 4 ml/kg is necessary, consult the pulmonoligist.

Minute Volume

Adjust the respiratory rate to achieve the desired minute volume as determined by calculations based upon BSA. Consult the pulmonologist to consider permissive hypercarbia or inverse ratio in a pressure control mode if MV cannot be maintained within the following parameters:

- Rate $\geq$ 35

- V_T < 4ml/kg or > than 6 ml/kg

- PIP $\leq$ 30 cm H_2O

- Pplateau $\leq$ 30 cm H_2O

Fine-Tuning Parameters

Set the airway pressure alarm at 35 cm H_2O to limit the maximal airway pressure to 30 cm H_2O. To facilitate and ease WOB, consider using autoflow and a low flow trigger. If the requisite V_T is less than 6 ml/kg IBW, make regular attempts to increase V_T in increments of 1 ml/kg IBW to achieve 6 ml/kg. If the patient is receiving 6 ml/kg, attempt to reduce the inspiratory time to achieve an I:E ratio of 1:3.

Oxygenation

By definition, due to the nature of the disease, normal oxygenation is not possible; therefore, the oxygenation goal in ARDS/ALI is to maintain a PaO_2 of 55 to 80 mm Hg or SpO_2 at 88 to 95%. Also due to the nature of the disease, this will generally require levels of PEEP greater than the 5 cm H_2O generally applied to emulate anatomical PEEP.

Table of FiO2 versus PEEP

Consider the following combinations of F_iO_2 to PEEP to achieve the oxygenation goal. It is not necessary to obtain an ABG with every change; SpO_2 readings are sufficient. However, if a PaO_2 is available, it of course supersedes the SpO_2.

F_iO_2 %:	30	40	40	50	50	60	70	70	70	80	90	90	90	100
PEEP:	5	5	8	8	10	10	10	12	14	14	14	16	18	20-24

Plateau Pressure

Another goal is to maintain plateau pressures within certain parameters (Pplateau $\geq$ 25 cm H_2O and $\leq$ 30 cm H_2O). As such, the Pplateau should be checked at least Q4, as well as after each change in PEEP or V_T.

- Pplateau > 30 cm H_2O, decrease V_T in 1 ml/kg increments to a minimum of 4 ml/kg.

- Pplateau < 25 cm H_2O and V_T < 6 ml/kg, increase V_T by 1 ml/kg increments until Pplateau > 25 cm H_2O or V_T = 6 ml/kg.

- Pplateau < 30 and breath stacking or dys-synchrony occurs, consider increasing V_T in 1 ml/kg increments to 7 or 8 ml/kg if Pplateau remains < 30 cm H_2O.

pH Parameters

Permissive hypercapnia is not uncommon in ARDS/ALI patients; thus the goal is to maintain a pH of 7.30 to 7.45. If acidosis fails below pH 7.30 and cannot be managed by the aforementioned ventilation parameters, consult the pulmonologist and consider $NaHCO_3$.

Chapter Eight
Ventilator Weaning

Weaning parameters are designed to move the patient safely toward liberation from ventilatory support. Each patient is different and thus will respond differently. Some require little to no weaning at all, while others may take days or weeks. In either case, once the underlining medical condition that provoked the need for mechanical ventilation is resolved, a reduction of ventilatory support should be considered with the goal of liberation from the ventilator. As such, the following guidelines might be helpful

Important Weaning Considerations

Several factors can be involved in the weaning process, especially for those patients who have been very ill. Therefore, before considering initiating the weaning process certain criteria must be considered.

Clinical Status

First we must verify that the underlying diseases process, which initiated the need for mechanical ventilation, is sufficiently resolved and that the patient is strong enough and able to maintain adequate ventilation and oxygenation for short periods of time.

Vital Signs

The patient's temperature should be < 102 Fahrenheit with hemodynamic stability, which is defined as:

- Normal heart rate.

- Absence of active myocardial ischemia.

- Absence of hypertension beyond patient's normal or systolic BP > 180.

- Absence of hypotension, systolic < 90.

- Absence of clinically important hypotension (i.e. no vasopressor therapy; or minimally, a therapeutically low-dose vasopressor such as dopamine or dobutamine < 5 micro g/kg/min).

Optional measurements would be:
- A-a DO_2 < 300 mmHg.
- Q_S/Q_T < 20%; and V_D/V_T < 60%.

However, unless the patient has suffered severe illness such as ARDS/ALI these measurements are seldom performed.

Basic Pulmonary Functions

The following criteria are generally considered vital weaning parameters. They are to be measured without ventilatory support.

- $V_T \geq 5$ mL/kg

- $VC \geq 10$ ml/kg (V_T x 2)

- RR 8 - 30 breaths per minute

- $V_E \leq 10$ L/min

- NIF $\geq$ -20cm H_2O

- RSBI < 100 (f/ V_T in L)

Oxygenation

Adequate oxygenation should be present. For the purpose of weaning, this is generally defined as $PaO_2/F_iO_2 > 150$-200 with PEEP $\geq$ 5- 8 cm H_2O or $SaO_2 \geq 92\%$ on $\leq 50\%$ FiO_2.

Exceptions can be made for chronic CO_2 retainers, wherein otherwise abnormal (slightly acidotic and hypoxemic) ABG values are considered acceptable: (e.g. pH $\geq$ 7.30 and $PCO_2 \leq$ 75, $SaO_2 \geq 88\%$). These values are accepted in this patient population because this is where they live. Even if their ABGs were normalized via ventilatory assistance, they would return to their abnormal values as soon as they are off the ventilator. So then, the goal is to achieve ABGs values that are normal for their chronic condition rather than values that are normal for normal lungs.

Spontaneous Breathing Trials

Once the appropriate criteria have been met, we initiate the weaning process by incorporating spontaneous breathing trials (SBT) via unassisted breathing. SBT differs from the spontaneous mode in that during SBT therapeutic levels of neither CPAP nor PS are employed. CPAP ≤ 5 cm H_2O and PS ≤ 5 cm H_2O are not considered therapeutic in that they merely serve to overcome the complications created by the endotracheal tube: i.e. the absence of anatomical PEEP provided by the epiglottis, and the restricted lumen through which the patient must breath.

Adequate spontaneous respiratory efforts must be assessed as well. For this the mechanical respiratory rate can be decrease by 50% for 5 minutes to detect the patient's spontaneous respiratory efforts. The ability to maintain an adequate minute volume without a dramatically increase WOB is at issue; thus a RR of 8 to 30.

Initializing SBT

The initial SBT should last from 1 to 5 minutes with the following parameters:

- Ventilator in spontaneous mode.
- FiO2 $\leq 50\%$.
- PS ≤ 5 cm H_2O.
- PEEP ≤ 5 cm H_2O.

Reassessment, based upon the aforementioned parameters, should occur at five minutes. If SBT fails, return the patient to the ventilatory support in use prior to SBT. Let the patient rest a minimum of 24 hours before attempting SBT again. Repeated the 1 to 5 minute SBT each day until the entire 5 minutes is tolerated.

Once a 5 minute SBT is tolerated, and the patient is able to maintain a $SaO_2 \geq 92\%$ with PEEP and $F_IO_2 \leq$ the settings used in previous session, proceed to prolonged daily SBTs lasting up to 30, 60, 90 and 120 minutes. Reassess the patient at each interval to determine SBT continuation or discontinuation.

When short-term ventilator patients (i.e. ≤ 24 hours, such as post anesthesia, or an acute fluid overload) meet the weaning criteria and tolerate SBT for 60 to 120 minutes, it is generally acceptable to proceed to immediate extubation.

Sustained Criteria During SBT

Stability must be maintained throughout all stages of SBT irregardless of the weaning mode. Failure to stay within these parameters is considered SBT failure and the patient should be returned to the support mode in use prior to attempted SBT.

- $V_T \geq 5$ mL/kg
- Respiratory Rate 8 - 35 breaths per minute
- $V_E \leq 10$ L/min
- RSBI < 100 (f/ V_T in L)

- BP Normal for patient

- HR > 120% of resting AM baseline lasting > 5 minutes

- Respiratory Rate > 35.

- SpO_2 <88%

- Two or more signs outward signs of respiratory distress, which indicate inward changes.

    ✓ Marked use of accessory muscles

    ✓ Abdominal paradox

    ✓ Diaphoresis and signs of anxiety

    ✓ Marked complaints of dyspnea

Occasionally it may be appropriate to repeat the trial after an appropriate intervention such as suctioning, analgesia, bronchodilation, or some other factor that might contributed to SBT failure. Once the SBT of 120 minutes is tolerated, assess patient to consider permanent ventilator liberation and extubation.

www.ingramcontent.com/pod-product-compliance
Lightning Source LLC
Chambersburg PA
CBHW070556290526
45790CB00002B/709